To God Be The Glory

To God Be The Glory

◆

Losing Weight and Gaining Power

Yemina D. Thomas

iUniverse, Inc.
New York Lincoln Shanghai

To God Be The Glory
Losing Weight and Gaining Power

iUniverse books may be ordered through booksellers or by contacting:

iUniverse
2021 Pine Lake Road, Suite 100
Lincoln, NE 68512
www.iuniverse.com
1-800-Authors (1-800-288-4677)

Because of the dynamic nature of the Internet, any Web addresses or links contained in this book may have changed since publication and may no longer be valid.

You should not undertake any diet/exercise regimen recommended in this book before consulting your personal physician. Neither the author nor the publisher shall be responsible or liable for any loss or damage allegedly arising as a consequence of your use or application of any information or suggestions contained in this book.

ISBN: 978-0-595-42723-9 (pbk)
ISBN: 978-0-595-68568-4 (cloth)
ISBN: 978-0-595-87054-7 (ebk)

Printed in the United States of America

Contents

Acknowledgements

First and foremost, I want to thank my Lord and Savior Jesus Christ because with out Him I would be lost. I also want to send lots of love to my awesome and supportive husband, Zach, you deserve an extremely heart felt thank you for believing in me through my press toward something new. No one else on this earth can lift me up the way you do. To my daughters Nyeta and Kimata, Mommy loves you more than words could ever say. Thank you to my Pastor, Byron L. Broussard, you are a truly nurturing spiritual father who found the time in the middle of all that you do, to share your heart with me and give me the nudge and inspiration I needed. I thank my family especially my mother for living a health conscious existence, you laid the foundation I needed and I love you. To my church family at The Love Center in Atlanta, GA and everyone who gave me a word of encouragement instead of a look of judgment, I thank you as well.

Preface

I wrote this book to reach those who feel like they are all alone and in need of help. Information on how to lose weight is always accessible to us but, rarely do we hear about the struggles of losing weight and the story behind those hurdles. Everyone needs some inspiration and motivation at some point in their lives. This little book is a testimony of how I was able to succeed in achieving a healthier lifestyle after many failed attempts. You will have the opportunity to see yourself in my struggles as well as my victories as you learn to attain your healthier lifestyle in this testimonial/journal. See how God has spoken and blessed me with restored health so that I would be able to say "To God Be the Glory". Use this book to take your quest for an improved relationship with God to a new place. Learn more about yourself through Him so that you can find the way to the path of consistency and a healthy quality of life.

1

The Biggest Weight of All

I am so glad to have the opportunity to share with you some of the things that God has shown me over the course of a year that have literally changed my life. It is my desire to broaden your perspective of the weight loss process. Before I begin I ask that you pray with me concerning the receptiveness of your heart, because beyond the physical changes that will be set into motion there will be an even greater change in your heart if you are truly open to what God has for you. You have to believe in God in order for any of this to be applicable to your life. This is intended to add to your walk with Christ, but there is never a wrong time to accept Him as your own. If you have not already received Christ as your personal Lord and Savior there is no better time than right now. This prayer of faith coupled with your sincere desire to know Him is a good start to a relationship with Christ.

Dear God, I confess that I am a sinner and ask you to forgive me and cleanse me from my sins. I want Jesus to come into my heart. I confess with my mouth that your son Jesus was born of a virgin, and raised from the dead. I thank you for your wonderful gift of salvation. Amen

The fact that you are reaching out to begin a change in your life says that you have encountered some issues that you can not resolve on your own. So let's begin by preparing our hearts to absorb and then seal all that the Lord will show us throughout this process.

God, I love you and I thank you for your awesome grace and mercy. You are my Lord and my Savior. You made me and you know me better than I know myself, help me to know the body you have placed me in. Lord, I need you to activate your spirits of discipline, sacrifice and consistency in me. Teach me about myself so that I may better serve You. In Jesus' name I pray. Amen.

There will never be two identical stories. I encourage you to write down your experiences in order to document your journey of improvement. Take a picture of yourself every other month as a tangible part of your testimony. I wish someone would have shared this tip with me because, each phase of weight loss seems to carry with it different characteristics. In my case the first few weeks were mostly a change in my face and neck. Later there was noticeable shrinkage of my waist and arms however; the most important change was the new found respect I have for myself. There isn't one formula for weight loss, but we will be consulting God's word therefore, you will receive customized instructions and reassurance. Use what you will read as a guideline for positive change. You can do anything you believe and you will not fail unless you decide to. *"I can do all things through Christ which strengthens me. Phil 4:13"* Roget's College Dictionary defines health as: sanity, soundness, vigor, vitality, strength, wholesome, clean and in shape. If someone were asked to describe you would any of these words be used? I hope that the words I have to share with you will escort you to the lost and found where you can recover and fortify these attributes to your character. It is torture to try to be physically healthy while your mental and spiritual state are neglected or damaged. I like to use an analogy that says that we all are flowers in God's garden. Each phase of our lives affects the way the plants grow. In this next chapter I will share with you the seeds that were sown to grow the insecurities concerning my body.

2

The Seeds

My story is not one of a woman who was once thin and athletic. I didn't just recently gain a few pounds due to the demands of life. I was a pudgy little girl who loved my granddaddy's cooking and I grew into a fat woman who never lost her bad habits and insecurities. I felt that being fat was cute, loveable, and comfortable. I felt that being heavy and less attractive than those around me made me a safe person to befriend. I guess now that I have learned more about myself, I realize that all I really wanted was the gratification of friendship and I was willing to compromise my appearance to have that in my life. This has become a life lesson I try to share with anyone who is struggling with their place in life whether weight is their challenge or not. Too often we are the cause of our own unhappiness while trying to please others and that simply does not add to the quality of our lives. As a teenager it was difficult for me to participate in some of the things I really wanted to do because I worried that other people would be focusing on my size and not my personality. In actuality I was slightly overweight, but the years of telling myself how fat I was and comparing myself to others had already taken its toll on my self image. My family would affectionately joke and make comments about my weight and I adjusted to hearing my peers tease me. I would pretend to be unaffected, but I was pierced every time someone made any reference to my size. It felt like I was being judged and defined by the very thing I disliked most. In response I abused the food to distract me from the discomforts of my insecurities. Like every other young girl I wanted to feel pretty and accepted yet, I created a wall within my heart that kept me in a tunnel because I couldn't handle being judged or rejected. Over time a minor inconvenience developed into an overwhelming problem. As the years went by my weight continued to increase. During my second pregnancy I reached my all time high of 270 pounds on a 5'5" frame. In the following months and years afterward I held steady between 250 and 225 pounds, stretching my body far beyond its limits for nearly four years after giving birth. I allowed my size to place limits on who I was and what I could do. If I stepped out of my zone to try something new people may have noticed and I did not want to draw any attention to myself. I began to take on the lifestyle of a seventy year old grandma instead of living the active life of a twenty five year old woman. I love to cook for my family and the feeling I get when they are all enjoying a meal that I have prepared is priceless. I would prepare large heavy meals daily and then spend hours in front of the television. One day I looked at a picture and I didn't recognize myself anymore. I honestly thought I was looking at a picture of someone else. My husband would always tell me how beautiful he thought I was and I doubted his sincerity, the problem was that I didn't feel beautiful. I thought that he was telling me those things out of routine. I tried to dress myself up to look like people I thought were attractive, and of course it did not help to improve my self image. I was at a transition point in my life and was apprehensive about the direction my life was going.

3

The Unexpected Gardener

The opportunity for change presented itself to me and my first instinct was to go further into my shell. God's timing is so divine and He used a friendly weight loss challenge within J.U.S.T (Jesus Ultimately Saves and Transforms) Sisters, the women's ministry at my church as the first step in making my initiative for change a true commitment. Even as I sit here sharing my story with you my heart is filled with mixed emotions. There is sadness after wasting so much time hiding when the solution was there for me all of the time and joy because I have accepted God's plan for my life and I am so grateful for his patience with me. I now make a conscious effort never to mistreat God's property again. "*Or do you not know that your body is the temple of the Holy Spirit who is in you, whom you have from God, and you are not your own? For you were bought with a price; therefore glorify God in your body and in your spirit, which are God's. 1 Corinthians 6:19–20*" I feel so relieved now that I have given myself permission to remove my shell and be who I truly am. My shell guarded me from receiving so many wonderful things from the people in my life and kept me from sharing myself with others. When you look at life from a shell it is actually a very lonely existence. Recognizing why I've done some things has given me a peace about where I stand today. I am so uncomfortable with being pretentious because I know that I am good enough and I don't have to mask myself anymore. I forgive everyone who said things that affected me in that way whether they intended to or not. I am focused on growing in Christ now and I am moving on to better things. I am now a woman who is vulnerable enough to share some very intimate issues yet, strong enough to survive the judgments that will come as a result. It is so crucial that we lie aside our finite way of viewing life and try to see things as God does. Your journey is for you as well as countless others so if you are open to be blessed you can truly be used to affect change.

If you are unhappy with your current weight don't waste another minute of another day. Life is too precious to waste and we can not take for granted the miracles God allows us everyday. We often miss out on blessings because we keep our minds preoccupied with the trivialities in life. I like to write out comparisons to help me when I just can't seem to get a grip on things. For instance, I may have a goal to lose five pounds for my birthday and then someone sends me a box of my favorite chocolates. My flesh would have me eat the box of chocolate without discretion however; I know that I will feel better about myself if I use discipline in order to reach my goal. Ultimately I will be better rewarded if I eat one chocolate and share the rest. I have to make the decision to do what is best for the long term. Don't shake your head and blame the devil because, God has a funny way of testing us at times. We are flesh and our lives will not be perfect but we can strive to live a life of balance and order instead of chaos.

Visualize yourself lending someone a top of the line luxury car with a lifetime supply of gas and oil. Now imagine that the person has borrowed your car only to abuse it and provide little or no maintenance to the car until it is returned. You would feel disrespected and used among other things. I believe that this is the way God sees us at times and it saddens Him. We misuse what is not really ours and we don't appreciate the gift that life is. As a child, whenever we visited someone else's home, my mother would always say that in some way, we should leave things better than we find them. I realize that I cannot improve on God's creation, but I can do my best to maintain myself at an acceptable level. I want to show my creator that I am appreciative of the vessel He has given me and the opportunities I have to use it for His glory. So often we look to God for more stuff and things and we are not even taking care of what He has already given us.

I have tried all kinds of diets, shakes, and pills and nothing ever gave me the results I was hoping for. At times, I even suffered from side affects, yet I continued to use different products because my faith was displaced. I was willing to tolerate diarrhea, nausea, and rashes and other discomforts for a chance at being thin. I didn't believe that I was capable of change and I hadn't even considered asking God for help. I was taking risks with my body and paying the cost physically as well as mentally. My self esteem sustained lasting damage with each unsuccessful attempt, and I became submerged deeper in feelings of insecurity, guilt and failure. I protected myself against experiencing my emotions by joking or commenting on my weight before anyone else could. I was my own worst enemy because I constantly abused myself emotionally in an attempt to project a confident self image to cover the depression I was drifting in and out of. I am not telling you this to make you feel sorry for me, instead I want you to understand the pain that attaches itself to complacency. I knew that I needed to change; however, I was afraid of the possible discomfort and inconvenience I would experience in unfamiliar territory. I pray that you are also able to see how awesome God is; He will repair weaknesses you are aware of as well as the ones you don't even see. Once I became saved I began to pray that God would just take this weight off of me and help me to control my over eating still I stayed overweight because I wanted God to erase years of damage with little to no work on my part. I wanted to use God as my personal wish master so that I could be like the people I thought were better and more attractive than I.

God first had to show me that I was worthy of better because He created and loves me. He began to water, feed and remove the weeds that were hiding my issues. We teach our children that "God don't make no junk" and somehow that gets lost as we age and tamper with His creation. God doesn't make mistakes, but people do and we need His guidance to recover from the messes we create. My intentions are now tied to His word and His heart and not my own selfish and absurd motives. I am good enough because of His spirit in me rather than in comparison to anyone else. For God so loved the world that He gave His only begotten son; that means that we are all precious to God, enough to require such an awesome sacrifice to save our lives. Now that I have opened my heart I have seen tremendous results in my life and I am encouraged to continue to press toward my goal of overall health. There are no secrets or tricks to losing weight in this book because I am seeking to help you develop a plan for your life so that you will truly grow and never need to revert to old habits. God led me out of a life long habit of unhealthy eating and activities so He can and will do the same for you. My desire is to successfully reach my goal using only what God has revealed to me about myself. When people ask me how I was able to get where I am I want to be able to say "To God Be the Glory". I am not for or against diets or weight loss programs; I realized that God has set a different path for me. If you are a part of a program this information is still for you because we are dealing with life change in more than one dimension. I urge you to take from this what applies to your life and hold the reserve information to possibly bless someone else. The new habits you adapt will help you keep the weight off once you have reached your goal.

Sometimes we are simply lacking in the ability to be truthful with ourselves. In my case, prior to the challenge I had become more physical still I could not lose weight consistently. Then the problem was that I was ignoring my addiction to butter and sugar. I would go for a wonderful walk in the park and then stop by the grocery store for a donut or a snickers bar. I finally had to face myself and change my practice of habitual deceit. I was not doing myself a favor and I would never see the results I desired until I paired my new activity with healthier eating. My first step toward a healthier lifestyle was to take inventory of my life. Just because no one saw you eat a box of cookies doesn't erase the fact that it happened. Ask yourself what it is that you are unhappy with, as well as, what you are happy with concerning your health? It is important to know this before you begin because you will want to acknowledge the things that are positive and focus your energy on the things that need the most attention. One of the positives could be that you are open to and ready for change. No one is motivated when they feel like a total failure; we just need to improve our lifestyles so that we are more in line with God's word. The truth will set you free so be honest with yourself, because God already knows all about you He's just waiting for you to wake up. Most of us have been in an unhealthy pattern for so long that we will practically be reborn into this new lifestyle, but that is okay. God knows that sometimes we will have to start over in order to grow properly, and in starting over you have to recommit yourself to doing things His way. "*As newborn babes, desire the sincere milk of the word, that ye may grow thereby: 1 Peter2:2*". I believe that God grants us new beginnings because we need to capture the zeal and excitement people possess when they discover a new passion. This is a very intimate process so be specific and genuine when talking with God about your life change. There is no issue too small or too large for God to handle so give Him everything that comes into your heart. Please use the page provided to list your top five negatives and positives. Set your target weight, there is a guide in the back of this book to help you. I am asking for five of each aspect because most people are able to list tons of negatives and only a few positives. We don't want to begin with an unbalanced or badgered mind frame.

POSITIVES

1. _____

Why? _____

2. _____

Why? _____

3. _____

Why? _____

4. _____

Why? _____

5. _____

Why? _____

NEGATIVES

1. _____

Why? _____

2. _____

Why? _____

3. _____

Why? _____

4. _____

Why? _____

5. _____

Why? _____

☺TARGET WEIGHT _____
CURRENT WEIGHT _____

4

My Toughest Weed

You made it this far, why not keep going, give yourself a moment to take a deep cleansing breath, wipe the sweat from your brow or the tears from your eyes because it will only get better from here. I realize that each person's daily schedule is different and some are more challenging than others. We are making a life change and it requires the elimination of all excuses. My spiritual father has always taught his children that if you want something you've never had before then you have to do something you've never done before. Wherever you see or feel any conflict, know that you have prayed and that God has heard you. *"Being confident of this very thing, that He who has begun a good work in you will complete it until the day of Jesus Christ; Phil 1:6"*. He will provide a way for you to reach your goals. God words are full of promise and they are the only promises that are guaranteed to come to pass. Each of us has been placed on this earth for a set purpose so we all have access to everything we need to do what we were placed here to do.

My personal challenge has been procrastination. It is such a clever way to avoid doing the things we know we should. Procrastination keeps us from having to out right say "no" to something, instead we can say later and so often later turns into never. I am a wife, mother, and active church member so there is never a shortage of things I could be doing. However, in order to break the hold that delay had placed on me I needed to learn to organize and prioritize as much as I possibly could. My health had to fit into my daily agenda at some point or I would continue to suffer as a result. Being important in my own life was so hard for me because it is my nature to nurture and care for everyone around me. I felt extremely guilty and selfish at first because it had been so long since I'd spent my time caring for me. Even in the time I had set aside for myself my mind would wonder about other people and things in my life. One day while I was on the treadmill, I realized that I was sabotaging my own workout because I would distract myself with the television or thinking about what I was going to do once I was finished. I made up my mind to make that time about God and I. Before I knew it what would normally have been a twenty minute session had turn into an hour. My body felt rejuvenated and my heart was so content because I could feel that God was pleased with my decision. Taking time to care for myself does not negate the love and concern I have for the people in life, it actually makes me more able to pour into them without going physically and spiritually bankrupt.

I don't have time! Let's deal with one of the most common excuses we use for our unhealthy habits. Everyone, no matter who you are, can find thirty to fourty five minutes a day to do some form of exercise. Most of our normal daily activities can be turned into dual purpose activities easily. For example, while watching TV you

can also do sit ups, stretches, jog in place or even jump-
ing jacks. Pack a nice, healthy meal and walk to a peace-
ful spot during lunch or play a game with your children
my girls and I enjoy the hula hoop which is good for the
waistline as well as the soul. Also, try taking the stairs
instead of the elevator, put on your favorite praise CD
and dance around the house or literally walk around the
mall by strolling around the outside. If you're stuck in
traffic then use that time to work on your abdominals
by contracting the muscles for 20–30 seconds at a time.
This is a good way to start incorporating some activity;
however, as you progress I encourage you to challenge
your body and allow the routines to gradually increase
in intensity. As you can see there are lots of ways to get
in some physical activity throughout the day especially
if it is a priority for you. There are so many resources
available to us to help us find new and exciting ways to
strengthen our bodies. If you start this journey with
exercise you will see better results and challenge your
body more often. I started out as a loner, exercising to
video tapes in my family room and as I saw my endur-
ance building I gained the confidence to venture out
and the need to exert myself more. I have discovered
that I prefer to exercise with a partner or in a class set-

ting because it satisfies the slightly competitive nature I never knew I had. I tend to push myself just a little harder when I am with a group of people who have a common goal. It feels so good to hear someone encourage me to press on and vice versa. Some things are for a certain season in your life, and I believe that for that brief period, I was supposed to be secluded so that I could establish myself. We can't be afraid to switch things up from time to time. Our bodies have the ability to become accustomed to a repeated activity so that it loses it effectiveness. Variety is important so that you can get the most out of your workout. You may feel somewhat overwhelmed with all of the new changes you are putting into place, but nothing worthwhile comes with out a high price and eventually it will all become a part of you. Don't skip your work out just because you are a little sore or stiff. Once you warm your muscles you will be able to have a productive exercise session. If you feel sore after a workout, soak in a warm Epsom Salt bath then give your body a good stretch afterward. Your muscles will eventually get used to the stretching and growth. If an activity becomes boring try something new. We have to get our bodies moving and our heart rates up on a daily basis in order to firm and tone our bodies as the pounds come off. We are talking about preventative medicine here. I would burn my poor husband out requesting a back massage on a weekly basis because of the pressure the extra weight put on my back. I wanted to treat the symptom and not the source, as I exercised I strengthened my core muscles which alleviated much of the back pain I was experiencing. It feels so much better to have my husband massage my back because he wants to and not because I am begging him to. Exercise is also proven to boost brain power, improve sleep, relieves PMS symptoms, lower risk of heart disease, high blood pressure, and osteoporosis. Honestly, there will be days when you absolutely do not want to exercise, but don't you give up. You only need to exercise four to five days a week for a minimum of thirty minutes. Time is valuable so we must learn to budget it as well. Be sure to incorporate stretching into each workout to get the most out of any exercises you do. The motivation for change is a key element because if you are doing this to prove something to others or satisfy your own flesh you will eventually quit. However, when your motivation is greater than your small way of thinking you will allow yourself the feeling of empowerment when you press past your flesh to do something good for you. *"The soul of a lazy man desires, and has nothing; but the soul of the diligent shall be made rich. Proverbs13:4"*. What are your plans for developing a more active lifestyle? Make a commitment to yourself and write down your feelings toward that commitment.

5

Turning the soil

Here's where the list of the five negatives from page six comes in handy. Every plant pulls a significant amount of nutrients from its soil therefore, it is important to supply ourselves with quality nutrition. Of course, no one develops bad habits overnight; therefore, we can not expect to change them that way. We can however create an environment for ourselves that is conducive to our desired changes. Everyone can benefit from modifying their intake of salt, processed sugar, and simple carbohydrates. I have already confessed to being a sugar and butter junky so I'm not telling you about what I've heard but about what I know. Don't try to transform yourself instantly rather make small adjustments and gradually add to them as you become more comfortable. It will be a challenge to replace the habit of snacking on potato chips or cookies on a regular basis with snacking on whole grain crackers, fruits or fresh vegetables with dip. When choosing your snacks select unrefined foods as opposed to refined foods which are foods that have been processed. Refined foods do not retain as many of the vitamins and minerals we need. Are you still there? I am not saying that you can never have these things again; I am simply asking you to limit them. I find that keeping a healthy snack in my car or purse saves me from eating the convenient cheap snacks I would gravitate toward otherwise. If you are cost conscious like me you will want to plan your snacks ahead of time because impulse buying is not a good practice and healthier conveniently packaged foods are often priced a little higher. I believe that God has designed us so that we can eat as many fruits and vegetable as we would like without concern. My interpretation is that if God intended for the majority of our diet to be greasy, salty or sugary foods, He would not have placed man in a garden full of fruits, nuts, and vegetables. *"And the Lord commanded the man, saying, "Of every tree of the garden you may freely eat; Genesis 2:16"* Call me crazy if you like, this is the reasoning behind my practice of eating vegetables as my main dish and meat as a side. Try to stick with eating healthier for five to six days each week so that you can reward yourself over the next one to two days. You must consciously implement the moderation rule in your splurges especially with high fat/calorie foods. Once you know better you have to do better. *"By pride comes nothing but strife, but with the well-advised is wisdom. Proverbs 13:10"* As adults we cannot be forced to change, but if you know that you should be living a healthier life and you choose not to take action then you are responsible for consequences that come as a result of your decision.

Okay, now that we've made some practical changes in the snack drawer we can move on to the more intimidating task of planning our three major meals. Each person's meal planning criteria will vary, please refer to the charts in the back of the book to get a rough estimate of how many calories you should aim for each day.

In the beginning you should write down everything you eat throughout the day in order to create a mirror where you can see your strengths and weaknesses clearly. After a few weeks you probably will not need to use the journal any more but, keep it handy because it may serve as a pat on the back when you look back to see how your eating habits have improved. This was particularly enlightening for me because, I never knew that I was a full grown female "Mikey" or the clean up lady. When I forced myself to write down EVERYTHING, I noticed that I was eating what added up to about one extra meal a day just by finishing off the food that my children would leave on their plates. I was raised to eat everything on your plate and I carried that into adulthood. It would honestly bother me to see food go into the trash whether I was still hungry or not. I could not prepare a snack for my girls without tasting it. That mirror exposed some very ugly things, but I am glad to have uncovered them so that I can deal with them. Once I opened my eyes to that behavior I made a conscious decision to nip that in the bud. That was a major step for me in gaining self control.

Breakfast is very important so even if you're not a breakfast person force yourself to have at least a piece of fruit for breakfast and then have a healthy snack about two hours later. I have never been one to purposely skip a meal so my challenge was to make better food choices for breakfast. I had to cut back on the pancake and sausage days and add a variety of foods to my menu. If you take that word and break it down essentially "break" "fast" means that you are breaking the seven to eight hour fast your body went through during your sleep hours. If you have ever fasted, you know that eating greasy or salty foods immediately after a fast can irritate your stomach and leave you feeling a little ill. I try to keep this in mind when I plan out my breakfast because I don't want to have to pay that price for rest of day. Breakfast is a key element in jump starting your metabolism. Breakfast or lunch should contain a complex carbohydrate and be your largest meal of the day because this is when your metabolism is at its peak and you have the rest of the day to turn that food into energy. Carbohydrates are not the enemy, Thank God! In fact we need them for sustained energy throughout the day. However, we should be informed about which carbohydrates are better for our bodies. There are two basic forms of carbohydrates, complex and simple. Simple carbohydrates are simple sugars, sucrose (table sugar), fructose (fruit sugar) and lactose (milk sugar). Complex carbohydrates take longer for our bodies to breakdown and they are mostly found in vegetables, whole grains, and beans. Complex Carbohydrates keep us feeling full for longer periods of time.

6

Your Timing

Dinner should be eaten at least 2–3 hours before bedtime this will give you a more restful night sleep and you will not interfere with your resting metabolic rate. You will find that you will eat about six to seven times per day which may seem like a lot but in order for your body to have the energy to burn fat you have to eat. Eating smaller meals more often also keeps your blood sugar levels stable so that you don't experience the highs and lows of being hungry. It also speeds up our metabolism because, it is constantly in use. As we get older our metabolism slows a bit anyway so this is my way of taking action against it. This is like a two fold blessing for me because I don't have to worry about being distracted by hunger and I don't have to binge in order to satisfy my appetite. We need food because our bodies convert it into energy and you want to avoid feeling sluggish. When you do not eat your body will go into what is called "starvation mode" where it holds on to all of its fat and water to preserve itself. Of course, no one is perfect and not everyday is routine so if you must have a late dinner try drinking a full glass of water before you eat a salad or a cup of soup. If you're still not satisfied after ten minutes have a cup of tea or a sugar free Jell-O cup.

It takes the brain about ten minutes to register when the stomach is full, so take the time to savor and thoroughly chew your food. Then give your brain that ten minutes, most likely you will feel full or you will convince yourself that you don't really need what you are craving anyway. Our lives have become so busy that we don't take the time to talk to our loved ones. I like to check in on everyone at the dinner table and just talk or laugh. By the time we're done that ten minutes has passed and I am free of the struggle. If you live alone take, this time to clean the kitchen or call a loved one on the phone you will get the same result. A human's stomach is only as big as his or her fist so it really doesn't take much to fill it. It may take a few weeks for your stomach to adjust to eating normal food portions because overeating can cause the stomach to stretch. As a woman who would eat not only her own dinner, but also the scraps of others I know exactly what I am talking about. I had gotten to a point where I could eat more than my husband who is not exactly a tiny man. I would feel so ashamed when everyone would get up from the table and leave me sitting there eating my second or third portion. As I began to cut back, my portions got smaller, and I surprised myself with the amount of food it really takes to satisfy my hunger. Be consistent with your portion control and your stomach will return to its appropriate size. When eating a meal don't be afraid to leave something on the plate, especially when dining out since restaurant portions are often too large specifically in the starch group. Don't throw away a week's worth of disciplined eating and exercise for an entire basket of bread sticks or a double portion of mashed potatoes. A common misconception is that when you have a good exercise session you are then allowed to have more calories and fat. This is simply not true, because while you are trying to lose pounds you will need to stay within your calorie intake range. Trust that the same filling fruits and veggies that kept you going in the beginning will continue to serve their purpose. You will be able to have mini splurges more often once you gain a reasonable amount of self control and have come close to your target weight. This change is for the rest of your life. Don't look at what you're giving up, instead, look at what you will gain. You have the power to use self control by literally cutting the temptation and requesting an extra plate or a carry out box when dinning out. Cut your portions in half and share with others at your table or have some for lunch the next day, you'll either make your dollar go a little further or give your table mates a variety of things to sample. It may seem like a small victory, but I am so pleased not to be the one taking the excess food from all of the plates on the table home with me for a late night snack. I have grown out of that hording behavior and I don't have to worry about that kind of embarrassment again.

There really aren't any bad foods if you learn moderation. If we consume more of the foods that are highly beneficial to our bodies then there will be less room for the foods that have less nutritional value. After suffering with them for years, I received some relief from chronic allergies as a result of changing my diet which has truly added to the quality of my life. As you gradually cut back on eating processed foods and salts, you will develop a preference for healthier foods.

7

Water:
An Absolute Necessity

One of the most important things you can do is to add more water to your regimen. It cleanses your system of toxins, it regulates your body temperature, it helps you to digest your food, it hydrates the skin and muscles and it aids in the breakdown of fat cells. Water is also a natural diuretic which helps to control water retention. Too much salt, on the other hand, can cause your body to hold water so be mindful of your salt intake as well. Soon you will be able to work your way up to a standard of eight to ten glasses of water each day. Get ready to visit the restroom a lot more often until your body adjusts to taking in the extra water. For those who do not enjoy the taste of water I suggest adding some lemon juice or drinking it with a straw. Also, eat more fruits and vegetable that are high in water content. One of my rules is that I must drink more water than any other liquid. This was a personal goal for me because my husband and I both love to drink sweetened iced tea which kept me from drinking the water I needed. I often carry a 64 ounce thermos of water with me so that I can drink from it when I want to and I fill it twice a day giving me a total of 128 ounces of water. There are days that I am not able to drink the full 128 ounces so I treat each day as a new start and I aim to reach that goal the next day. God grants us brand new mercies everyday which mean that He is not looking to punish us for every mistake we've made. If God can forgive you why can't you forgive yourself? One of things I am learning from this process is how to bounce back. One mistake is not the end of the world for me unless I allow it to have more power than it should. I feel that if I never slip and fall then I won't be aware of the things I need to avoid in the future. Set backs are temporary yet, the life lessons I receive as a result of them will last forever. In life we go through processes in order to reach new levels in God, this is no different. Remember, this is your personal testimony about how God rewards obedience and discipline. Did you find any of the information applicable? Summarize the points that stood out for you to make them personal. I am sharing my story with you in order to help you build your own.

8

Look Ma

Hang in there and things will begin to turn around. In the beginning you will go through what I like to call the "look Ma no hands phase" where there is rapid weight loss due to the elimination of water weight. Rejoice, every achievement is worthy of being celebrated, still I urge you not to let this entice you into complacency. Now is not the time to have an ice cream party, you must stay focused on your goal. The first five pounds I lost was an extremely emotional accomplishment for me. When I stepped on the scale I was elated especially since I used to avoid the scale like the plague. I had never lost five pounds in less than two weeks before and this accomplishment only launched me further into my commitment to live healthy. My faith was also put into perspective because I knew that God would prove Himself, I just didn't realize it would happen so quickly. Originally, I had set a goal to lose thirty pounds because it seemed to be so far from where I was. My mind set still had not been fully broadened so all I wanted then was to get out of the two hundreds. Once I lost the thirty pounds I reevaluated my goal, by then I had learned to really push myself and I knew that I could go further. Over the next few months I was able to lose an additional twenty five pounds. I am now at a point where my focus is to lose inches instead of pounds. My goal has become to build muscle which weighs more than fat causing me to be heavier at times.

Let's not forget that as we focus on our bodies we can not neglect who we really are and that is the spirit inside the flesh. Find out what God has to say to you through His word through this book and your own exploration in Him. Gaining spiritual health has been the most rewarding aspect of this process for me because I feel as though I am stretching and growing beyond the box I had placed myself in. Balance is so important to me because it represents wholeness for me. I have become more conscious about paying attention to each aspect of my life because they all represent some part of who I am and I want to be complete. I don't want to be physically fit and spiritually wrecked so I have to feed my soul what it needs as well. My Pastor has been speaking on total stewardship for some time now, and much of that is tied to having a healthy spirit so I cannot be inattentive to mine. I knew that I could not hide my weight issues from the world, but I could disguise the issues I was dealing with in my spirit. God sees and knows my faults so I felt so foolish when I realized that I had essentially been putting on a bad production with some of the worst acting ever. We invest in the things that are important to us because we find them valuable. Trust that your spirit is a treasure to God therefore its worth is immeasurable. Imagine a mansion with beautiful architecture and perfect landscaping on the outside and on the inside you find faded curtains, torn linoleum and plastic furniture. Would you find it as attractive as one that is fabulous on the outside and even more gorgeous once you open the doors to see sparkling chandeliers, marble floors and satin drapes? *"I beseech you therefore brethren, by the mercies of God, that you present your bodies a living sacrifice, holy, acceptable to God, which is your reasonable service. And do not be conformed to this world, but be transformed by the renewing of your mind, that you may prove what is that good and acceptable and perfect will of God. Romans 12:1–2"*. The Lord is above all others and He deserves my very best. He knows that I cannot be perfect but He wants to use me as an example to the world of how His spirit makes me extraordinary. This is God's vision for all of us, to be Holy and healthy from the inside out.

9

Tying up loose ends

We have gone through the importance of portion control and water consumption. Now it's time to free your mind and try some different foods. We are now eating to live; therefore, we have made a conscious decision to consume foods that not only taste good but satisfy our body's need for nutrients. Once again, my mom knew exactly what she was doing when she'd give me that giant glass of orange juice when I caught a cold. Talk about multi tasking! In addition to its immune boosting properties, Vitamin C is also needed to keep your heart, eyes, teeth, joints, bones, muscles, and skin healthy. You can also find tons of Vitamin C in bell peppers, broccoli, cauliflower, kiwi and strawberries. There is a war of muscle versus fat going on so we have to help the muscle push the fat out of our way by providing ample potassium. Celery, a baked white or sweet potato, kiwi, cherries, mushrooms, and the ever faithful banana all contain moderate supplies of potassium. Muscles also need protein so we want to be sure to eat lean proteins such as fish, poultry, beans, dairy, or soy. This is so important for me because all of the years I had spent overweight had stretched my skin and caused me to lose muscle mass so that as I lost my weight I found a new struggle in trying to build muscle. I addition to making sure that I get enough protein I now use light weight lifting to rebuild my muscles and tone my body. Adding more fiber to our diet is crucial because, most people don't get enough fiber. One bowel movement per day is normal but we are not eliminating enough of what is essentially body garbage. The goal is to eat about six small meals and include fiber so that our bodies will take out the trash at least twice daily, now that's a well oiled machine! Think of a newborn baby, every time food goes into the baby shortly afterward something comes out, this is the way God designed us. Often adding fiber to your diet can cause some excess bloating especially in the beginning so to combat the gas and bloat try raw almonds, cinnamon, ginger or juices which have chemicals that release stored fat and toxins. Also, Chamomile and peppermint teas have become a staple in my home because they aid in proper food digestion. I have been blessed to have a mother who is a colon hydro therapist among other things. This process proves to be exceptionally helpful in helping the body eliminate the toxins that tend to build up over time in the colon. It's like pushing a restart button on your body because you feel like you are starting over with a clean slate. As you lose weight the toxins that were being held in your fat cells will be released and you will need to flush your system. Think of this as the clean up after the remodeling.

10

The Light You Share

I am creating a legacy by living a healthier life. I was so focused on committing to my change that I didn't even realize the effect it was having on my family. Making simple changes in the way I prepared meals for my family and providing them with better snacking options caused my husband to lose over 10 pounds effortlessly. My daughters began to try new foods and became more interested in exercise. Knowing that my family is benefiting from my life change has been a tremendous blessing to me and it only makes me want to push harder. It is more powerful to actually see a rainbow than it is to be told of one. Now I see that I am a role model for my children in more ways than I imagined. I don't want my children to grow up without respect for how God intended us to use our bodies. I feel that I am sowing seeds into their lives that will prove fruitful even once they've formed families of their own. They may not always be thrilled with options I give them, but I know that they will eventually appreciate what I have done for them out of pure love. God is blessing me so that I can bless someone else and I feel so privileged to be trusted with that responsibility.

God is ultimately in control. He allows us to make choices, and we should use those choices to prove that we have received His spirit of discipline. So when you find yourself at a birthday party, night out or even Thanksgiving Dinner remain confident with the choices you make and you will feel a sense of accomplishment and triumph over what used to be an issue for you. You may even bless the life of someone else without even trying, now isn't God awesome! Others are often watching your steps even closer than you.

During those busy times in your life when you have to stop at a fast food restaurant don't take the all or nothing approach. Try a child sized meal because those are the portions that actually fit more realistically into a stomach the size of a fist, or a grilled chicken sandwich with a side salad. The first time I used this strategy I was at lunch with my husband, and I ordered a child's meal after he had ordered his meal and up graded the fries and drink to an extra large. We sat down at the table to eat and I felt like such a lady as we ate our lunch that day because I wasn't eating portions that matched his and would make me feel guilty later. There is always a way to make healthier choices even when your options are limited. If you fall off of the healthy horse don't be afraid to jump back on immediately. The ride may get bumpy but, you have the power to tame that horse. *"Behold, I am the LORD, the God of all flesh. Is there anything too hard for me? Jeremiah 32:27"* God is greater than any obstacle you may encounter so lift your challenges to Him.

As adults we can be set in our likes and dislikes, give your palate a chance to adjust to some of the new flavors you'll encounter by reintroducing them at least 2–

3 times. After that if you still don't care for something it probably isn't for you. Be brave enough to try a new food and then, revisit this page to write about your experience? It may bless someone else to hear your story or it may be just plain funny. One of my comical experiences with trying something new happened when I tried soy nuts for the first time. There was a sale on them at the grocery store. I am usually very cautious about new things, but I guess the sale price impaired my judgment. Nevertheless, I bought a huge carton of them and began to snack on them in the car and discovered that they reminded me of cardboard. Until this experience I had never come across a nut that I didn't like, but the soy nuts just didn't seem to be for me. I tried them again the next day with some raisins and the taste did not change. I felt so guilty for buying all of those soy nuts and then wasting them but let's get real; no one is going to eat over a pound of something that tastes like the box it came in. This was one time where my frugal nature was overridden by my need for flavor.

11

Trust in Him

This process is all about growth because you will lose pounds and inches but you stand to gain so much more. You started this with God so stay here with Him. Once you reach or become very close to your healthy weight don't let the opinions and comments of others get you off track. As I began to lose more weight people would say to me, "Okay that's it, you don't need to lose another pound". This made me feel so self conscious about my appearance. Did I look sick? And had I gone too far? I would stand in the mirror and ask myself these questions. I wondered what they were seeing because I still saw a need to continue to lose. I had to come to grips with the fact that even though they meant no harm I was allowing them to interfere with what God is doing with me. I understand that it is difficult for those who knew me when I wore a size 22 to see me at a size 8. I found comfort in Psalm 37:5 where it says "commit your ways to the Lord, Trust in Him and He shall bring it to pass." God was testing me to see if my heart lined up with what my mouth was saying. I needed to decide whether being a people pleaser would produce a greater reward than being obedient to God and the answer was a resounding "NO". I had to prove that my commitment to Him was unwavering and that I trusted Him to bring this process full circle. Others may mean well, but above all I trust in God. Death and life are in the power of the tongue Proverbs 18:21. So speak life into your own situation so that you are not dependant on others to do so. Be encouraged at all times whether people acknowledge you or not. Let your motive to please God and not to seek the approval of others.

My changes were kept undercover until I grew to a place where I was secure enough to risk being judged by other people. I had lost some weight, but not enough for an outsider to really recognize so I kept it between God and I and that was enough for me. Eventually, people began to ask me how I had lost weight and by then I had experienced Him enough to know how to answer them. I know what God has spoken into my life throughout this process and no one in this world can take that from me. Good health requires life long effort so never stop seeking ways to better your own self. I pray that what I have shared with you has motivated you to be a better steward over the life that you have been blessed with. Our past experiences, whether good or bad, are our testimony so I encourage you to use them to help someone else embrace better health. If God doesn't get the glory then who does? We are on a mission not to be vain, but to put ourselves in a position to be used in the kingdom. Share this with someone who is stuck in the pattern you have now left behind. As believers, we represent Christ not only in what we say, but also in our actions and our appearance. Health translates into power which is a basis for conquering challenges in your life.

The kingdom of God is a dynamic force and we must have standards above those of the secular world. If we are bogged down with extra weight on our bodies and spirits how can we be swift to take action for His kingdom. Take a minute to think about how main stream entertainers put several hours a day into their exercise routines. They hire personal trainers to keep their bodies fit and they employ nutritionists to design specific diets for their bodies. All of this is a part of their marketing strategy. They realize that they will gain the support of their fans by making their lifestyle as attractive as possible. How will we win souls for Christ if we are perceived to be lazy and sedentary? I don't want to be the stereotypical Christian who is so caught up in being "holy" that they are no earthly good. For the record high cholesterol, diabetes, clogged arteries and high blood pressure are not what God intended for us. Our work is here on earth so we need to give our spirit transporters a tune up and get them moving. Let's step up our game and disprove the myth that once you're saved your life becomes dull and boring. My focus is not to make every believer into a runway model; instead I hope to motivate those who desire change to reach a healthy individual body weight. These charts are merely a guideline; I realize that individuals will differ due to different factors. Take the body that was misused by sin and turn it over to God for a total transformation. Are you ready to receive what God has for you?

12

Guidelines

WOMEN'S WEIGHT CHART

Height	Small Frame	Medium Frame	Large Frame
4'10"	102–111	109–121	118–131
4'11"	103–113	111–123	120–134
5'0"	104–115	113–126	122–137
5'1"	106–118	115–129	125–140
5'2"	108–121	118–132	128–143
5'3"	111–124	121–135	131–147
5'4"	114–127	124–138	134–151
5'5"	117–130	127–141	137–155
5'6"	120–133	130–144	140–159
5'7"	123–136	133–147	143–163
5'8	126–139	136–150	146–167
5'9'	129–142	139–153	149–170
5'10"	132–145	142–156	152–173
5'11"	135–148	145–159	155–176
6'0"	138–151	148–162	158–179

MEN'S WEIGHT CHART

Height	Small Frame	Medium Frame	Large Frame
5'2"	128–134	131–14	138–150
5'3"	130–136	133–143	140–153
5'4"	132–138	135–145	142–156
5'5"	134–140	137–148	144–160
5'6"	136–142	139–151	146–164
5'7"	138–145	142–154	149–168
5'8"	140–148	145–157	152–172
5'9"	142–151	151–163	158–180
5'10"	144–154	151–163	155–176
5'11"	146–157	154–166	161–184
6'0"	149–160	157–170	164–188
6'1"	152–164	160–174	168–192
6'2"	155–168	164–178	172–197
6'3"	158–172	167–182	176–202
6'4"	162–176	171–187	181–207

Source: www.healthchecksytems.com

GENERAL CALORIE REFERNCE

Food	Fat grams	Calo-ries	Car-bohy-drate	Pro-tein	Cho-les-terol	Satu-rated Fat grams
Whole Almonds 1oz	15	165	6	6	0	1.4
Apple Juice 1 c.	0	115	29	0	0	0
1/8 Apple Pie	18	405	60	3	0	4.6
1 c. sliced apples	1	125	32	0	0	0.1
Avocado	30	305	12	4	0	4.5
Egg Bagel	2	200	38	7	44	0.3
Banana	1	105	27	1	0	0.1
Beef Stew 1c.	11	220	15	16	10	4.3
Black eyed peas 1c.	1	190	35	13	0	0.2
Blueberries raw 1c.	1	80	20	1	0	0
Blueberry Muffins	5	140	22	3	45	1.4
Bologna 2 slices	16	180	2	7	31	6.1
Brownies w/ nuts	4	100	16	1	14	1.6

Food	Fat grams	Calo- ries	Car- bohy- drate	Pro- tein	Cho- les- terol	Satu- rated Fat grams
Broccoli raw 1 spear	1	40	8	4	0	0.1
Butter, unsalted ½ c.	92	810	0	1	247	57.1
Cooked cab- bage 1 c.	0	30	7	1	0	0
Cabbage, raw 1c.	0	15	4	1	0	0
Carrot cake w/frosting 1/8	21	385	48	4	74	4.1
Cantaloupe ½	1	95	22	2	0	0.1
1 Carrot	0	30	7	1	0	0
Cashews unsalted 1c.	63	750	37	21	0	12.4
1 Celery Stalk	0	5	1	0	0	0
Cheesecake 1/8	18	280	26	5	170	9.9
Cheesebur- ger	15	300	28	15	44	7.3
1 Chicken Breast fried	9	220	2	31	87	2.4

Food	Fat grams	Calories	Carbohydrate	Protein	Cholesterol	Saturated Fat grams
4 Chocolate chip cookies	9	180	28	2	5	2.9
Diet Cola	0	0	0	0	0	0
1 c. Collard greens Cooked	0	25	5	2	0	0.1
Corn Chips 1 oz.	9	155	16	2	0	1.4
Coffee black 6 oz.	0	0	1	0	0	0
1 egg fried	7	90	1	6	211	1.9
1 English muffin plain	1	140	27	5	0	0.3
Graham crackers 2	1	60	11	1	0	0.4
½ Grapefruit	0	40	10	1	0	0
10 grapes	0	35	9	0	0	0.1
Macaroni & Cheese baked	22	430	40	17	44	9.8
Oatmeal	2	145	25	6	0	0.4
Orange Juice 1c.	1	110	25	2	0	0.1
1 Pancake	2	60	8	2	16	0.5

Food	Fat grams	Calories	Carbohydrate	Protein	Cholesterol	Saturated Fat grams
Pecan Pie 1/8	32	575	71	7	95	4.7
1 slice Cheese Pizza	9	290	39	15	56	4.1
10 Pretzel sticks	0	10	2	0	0	0
Raisin Bran 1 oz.	1	90	21	3	0	0.1
Raisins 1c.	1	435	115	5	0	0.2
Rice, brown 1c.	1	230	50	5	0	0.3
Salmon baked 3 oz.	5	120	0	17	34	0.9
Choc. Shake	8	335	60	9	30	4.8
Strawberries 1 c.	1	45	10	1	0	0
Sunflower Seeds 1 oz.	14	160	5	6	0	1.5
Baked Sweet Potato	0	115	28	2	0	0
1c Vegetable Soup	2	70	12	2	0	0.3
Watermelon 1 c.	1	50	11	1	0	0.1

Food	Fat grams	Calo-ries	Car-bohy-drate	Pro-tein	Cho-les-terol	Satu-rated Fat grams
Whole wheat bread 1 slice	1	70	13	3	0	0.4
Wheat Thins Crackers 4	1	55	10	2	0	0.2
Yellow Cake w/frosting 1 piece	8	235	40	3	36	3
Low fat plain yogurt 8 oz.	4	145	16	12	14	2.3
Low fat yogurt w/fruit 8oz.	2	230	43	10	10	1.6

Source: www.caloriecountercharts.com

☺ Here is the general formula for better eating and a sample meal plan for one day. Drink 6–8 oz. of water before each meal. Once you have reached your target weight add an extra snack or two to your day. There are lots of different low fat/low calorie recipes that can be found in your favorite magazine or on the internet. Make collecting some healthier recipes a new project.

Breakfast = Carbohydrate (complex) + Protein or Vegetable

Lunch = Carbohydrate + 2 Vegetables or Protein + 2 Vegetables

Dinner = Protein + 2 Vegetables

Breakfast (with in one hour of waking up)
Egg white omelet with ½ cup of vegetables
1 slice of wheat toast with cream cheese
1 cup of coffee w/ low fat creamer
Or
8 oz. low fat yogurt
1 low fat granola bar
½ of an apple and a glass of carrot juice
Or

1 cup oatmeal with brown sugar or molasses
½ cup strawberries or blueberries
2 tbsp. pecans or walnuts
1 cup reduced fat or soy milk

A.M. Snack (about 2 hour later) ½ cup whole grain,
cereal w/1 c. low fat milk
Or 1 cup of seedless grapes
1 serving of Baked Tortilla Chips w/salsa
1 banana
Green tea

Lunch (about two hours later)
2 cups of vegetable soup
½ turkey sandwich
Handful of baby carrots
12 oz. Diet Coke Zero

P.M. Snack (2–3 hours later) Celery sticks
with peanut butter or low fat cream cheese
½ cup raisins and whole almonds unsalted

Dinner (2–3 hours before bedtime)
Large salad with flaxseed oil and Emeril's Salad Sea-

soning

Grilled chicken breast

¼ avocado or 2tbsp. sunflower seeds

Sugar Free Jell-O Cup

Or

Baked Fish with ½ cup brown rice and two of your favorite vegetables

Plus a low calorie or low fat dessert

• If you still are not satisfied add an additional healthy snack to your menu

SNACKS 100 CALORIES OR LESS

- 3 cups of light popcorn

- ½ apples with 1 Tbs. peanut butter

- 2 cups of baby carrots

- 1 granola bar

- Sugar Free Jell-O cup

- ¼ cup of Tofutti or Rice Dream

- 1 snack size chocolate bar

- ½ cup low or no fat frozen yogurt

- Apple dippers (McDonalds)

- Shredded lettuce rolled into in a slice of low fat turkey w/dressing for dipping

- Handful of peanuts or almonds

- ½ grapefruit

- Diet soda * all you want because it has no carbohydrates or calories

- Cucumber spears * all you can eat because cucumbers have a negative calorie effect

TONING EXERCISES
10–12 REPETITIONS EACH
Choose five exercises five days a week. Vary them to keep your workout fresh.

Arm Circles—Hold your arms straight out from your sides and rotate them ten time in each direction …

Twister—Stand up straight with your legs spread apart and hold your arms out from your sides and twist your upper body from left to right. Challenge your body by holding weight in your hands or holding the twist for 10 seconds on each side.

Toe Touches—Stand with your feet slightly apart. Slowly bend over as far as you comfortably can with your legs straight and hold the stretch for 5–10 seconds and repeat.

Trunk Benders—Stand with your feet shoulder width apart, and raise your arm up over your head toward the opposite hip. Slowly bend your torso sideways and hold the stretch for 10 sec.

Push Ups—Lie on the floor face down and place your hand just beneath your shoulders. Next lift your body up from the floor using your arms.

Calf Raises—Stand up on your toes as high as possible and pulse for 10 sec at a time.

Side Leg Lifts—Lie on your side with head supported by your hand and elbow and lift your leg as high as possible and then return it the starting position. Repeat for opposite leg.

Sit Ups—Lie on your back with your arms loosely behind the ears, bend your knees to a 90 degree angle bring your body to a sitting position.

Hamstring curls—Stand with your feet shoulder width apart and your stomach muscles tight. Pull your leg back at the knee so that your heel touches your buttocks. Alternate legs.

Squats—Stand with your feet slightly apart and you abdominals tight. Bend at the knees as if you are about to sit in a chair and then return to a standing position. For a challenge hold the squat position for ten seconds at a time before standing.

Bicep Curls—hold a comfortable weight in each hand. Hold your elbows close to your torso with your abdominals tight and then lift and lower. Remember to breathe during any exercise.

TARGET HEART RATE

The most acceptable form for determining you target heartbeat range and maximum heart beat rate is 220 minus your age. Mild exercise will produce 60–66 % of that and Moderate exercise will produce 67–73 %. For example, a man or woman who is 30 years old should have a heart rate of about 114–125 beats per minute during mild activities and 127–139 during moderate activity.

220 - _____ = _____
       age   max. heart rate

_____ x .60 = _____
max heart rate   mild heart rate

_____ x .67 = _____
max. heart rate   moderate heart rate

AVERAGE DAILY CALORIC INTAKE

Our bodies burn an average of ten times our body weight in calories each day with exercise added to the equation we are allowed a few more calories. For example, if a person weighs 160 pounds they are allowed about 1600 calories per day assuming that they are not participating in any extra physical activity. However, if that person takes a brisk thirty minute walk that burns 200 calories the caloric intake for that day increases to 1800. The objective is to burn more calories than we take in so think of exercise as a deposit into your calorie bank. The body has to burn about 3500 calories in order to lose one pound of fat. It should take about one week to lose 2–3 pounds.

13

The Big Picture

It is easy to become consumed with counting calories, pounds, or fat, but it is more important for you to simply be aware of what you are eating. You don't have to obsess over anything because you have what most don't—Faith. The information is there only to provide you with some parameters. Becoming overly selective about the foods you eat will cause you to feel negatively toward eating healthier. I am encouraging you to be your healthiest. This is not a diet it is a lifestyle change so there isn't a need to deprive your self of anything. A healthy lifestyle should not be full of the stress and pressure of monitoring pounds from day to day or isolating yourself from everything you enjoy for the sake of dieting. I face every day temptations like anyone else and there are times I win. There are also times when I give in. I can't tell you how many times a commercial has caused me to go the refrigerator to have a little something extra. However, as time goes on I've learned a few new ways to deter my impulse eating such as brushing my teeth, drinking a cup of tea or writing a note to myself. If no one else ever tells you that you're doing a great job you should. You have been there all along and you know how far you have come so write a nice note to yourself, you deserve it. I suggest that you discover some new interests or hobbies in order to avoid fulfilling every craving that comes along. Cravings are totally natural and once you have grown to the point where you can satisfy your cravings in moderation then give yourself a hand. However, while you cannot resist having a plate full of moist, delicious chocolate chip cookies you will need to find an outlet. This will also curb any emotional eating you may be doing as a result of being bored or stressed. I even joined the dance ministry at my church which is something I never would have had the confidence to do in the past. Perhaps you will pursue an interest that you never thought you would be able to or reintroduce yourself to an activity you used to enjoy.

Never measure your progress by someone else's. What God has for you is for you! Weight that comes off slowly is more likely to stay off. Your weight loss may not be as speedy as someone else's, keep in mind that we are pushing for long term success so we don't want to rush the process. It took about a year for me to lose sixty five pounds and I am still on my journey to reach my ultimate goal of seventy five pounds. Surround yourself with positive people. I was blessed to have other women at my church going through their weight loss process at the same time that I was. We encourage one another with compliments, tips or even just a big hug. Love like that will help to get you over any hurdles you may encounter. I knew that they sincerely wanted to see me succeed and it blessed me to have them in my corner. I love my "Chiseled Chosen". You don't have room for doubt and negativity in your life. God will do what He says. "*So shall My word be that goes forth from*

My mouth; It shall not return void, but it shall accomplish what I please, And it shall prosper in the thing for which I sent it. Isaiah 55:11."

Be proud of how far you have come and anticipate even greater results in the future. It was unrealistic for me to expect to look like someone who had lost ten pounds, but was only about fifteen pounds over weight when I had lost ten pounds at more than sixty pounds over weight. I allowed envy to spoil what was a great accomplishment because I didn't appreciate where God had brought me from. I now accept that there will always be someone taller or thinner than me, but I have to love who God has made me enough to believe in myself as well as the people around me. That is so easy to say, but so hard to do; however, the hardest tasks bring the greatest rewards. We all have the potential to reach our goals. God is not exclusive in His blessing; you can cause the hand of God to move with favor in your life by being diligent, obedient, and making sacrifices. The parable of the talents comes to mind when I think about what the Lord expects of me. Like the men in the parable of the servants and the talents. I am devoted to returning an increased blessing to God so that I can hear Him say, "Well done good and faithful servant". I do not want to be a disappointment to God because I took the blessings He has given me and kept them for myself. Nothing that happens in the life of a believer is for his or her benefit only. I am a light that God uses so that others may see Him more clearly. Despite the hurdles I face I will produce fruit. For some there may only be a few obstacles and for others it may seem as though issues and conflicts are constantly trying to hinder you. Be encouraged and stay focused no matter what comes your way. God will not allow you to go through more than you can handle, and you're stronger than you may think. He's there to fight battles for us that we are not strong enough to win on our own. I have learned to use conflict to pump up my spiritual muscles; I gain strength though it hurts at times. You have made a commitment to God to better yourself for His work. God has already promised you that He will be with you always. It is as if you literally have a body guard. God loves us and He only wants good things for us. The question we have to ask ourselves is are we as faithful and committed to Him as He is to us? Thank you for allowing me to impart to you what has transformed my heart, my body and ultimately my life. I

pray that I have left you feeling empowered and con-
victed about your walk. Here's an early Congratula-
tions!!! I just know you're gonna make it. God Bless!

978-0-595-42723-9
0-595-42723-5

www.ingramcontent.com/pod-product-compliance
Lightning Source LLC
Chambersburg PA
CBHW030349290526
45785CB00004B/1658